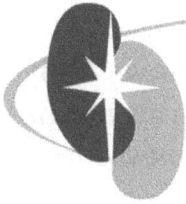

Renal Diet HQ IQ
Teaching You To Master Your Health

Dialysis: Treatment Options for the Progression to End Stage Renal Disease (ESRD)

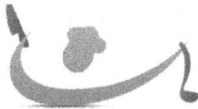

RENALDIET
HEADQUARTERS
BY HEALTHY DIET MENUS FOR YOU

Purpose and Introduction

What I have found through the emails and requests of my readers is that it is difficult to find information about a pre-dialysis kidney disease that is actionable. I want you to know that is what I intend to provide in all my books.

I wrote this book with you in mind: the person with kidney problems who does not know where to start or can't seem to get the answers that you need from other sources. This book will provide information that is applicable to a predialysis kidney disease.

Who am I? I am a registered dietitian in the USA who has been working with kidney patients for my entire 15 + years of experience. Find all my books on Amazon on my author page: http://www.amazon.com/Mathea-Ford/e/B008E1E7IS/

My goals are simple – to give some answers and to create an understanding of what is typical. In this series of 12 books, I will take you through the different parts of being a person with pre-dialysis kidney disease. It will not necessarily be what happens in your case, as everyone is an individual. I may simplify things in an effort to write them so that I feel you can learn the most from the information. This may mean that I don't say the exact things that your doctor would say. If you don't understand, please ask your doctor.

I want you to know, I am not a medical doctor and I am not aware of your particular condition. Information in this book is current as of publication, but may or may not have changed. This book is not meant to substitute for medical treatment for you, your friends, your caregivers, or your family members. You should not base treatment decisions solely on what is contained in this book. Develop your treatment plan with your doctors, nurses and the other medical professionals on your team. I recommend that you double-check any information with your medical team to verify if it applies to you.

In other words, I am not responsible for your medical care. I am providing this book for information and entertainment purposes, not medical diagnoses. Please consult with your doctor about any questions that you have about your particular case.

TABLE OF CONTENTS

PURPOSE AND INTRODUCTION 2

TREATMENT OPTIONS FOR KIDNEY DISEASE AND FAILURE 7

START WITH WHAT YOU CAN DO NOW (YOU ARE IN CONTROL)...7

AWARENESS 8

Known Risk Factors 8
Controlling Your Related Diseases 9
Medications Affect Your Kidneys.................................10

CHANGES AND PREVENTION.................................13

Talk To Your Doctor About Your Labs............................13
Change Medications If Needed....................................13
Follow A Healthy Low Protein Diet and Meal Pattern 13
Exercise – How Ever Much You Can 14
Track Your Progress...14

SEEK OUT INFORMATION FOR YOURSELF 17

Be Your Own Advocate 17
See the Right Doctor And Ask For Referrals If Necessary 17
What Can A Registered Dietitian Do? 18
Nurses Know A Lot – Just Ask!....................................18

STAGES OF LOSS 19

Denial 19
Anger 20
Bargaining 20
Depression 20
Acceptance 21

WHAT OPTIONS DO I HAVE?.....................................23

STAGE 5 ESRD 23
What Does Dialysis Do? 23
PERITONEAL DIALYSIS 24
What Is It? 24
How Does It Work? 25

What Does It Require? 26
Good Things About PD 26
Bad Things About PD 27
HEMODIALYSIS..29
What Is It? 29
How Does It Work? 29
In Center HD 30
Home HD..31
What Does It Require?...31
Good Things About HD 32
Bad Things About HD 32
TRANSPLANT 35
What Is It? 35
How Does It Work? 35
What Does It Require? 36
Good Things About Transplant 36
Bad Things About Transplant..37
NO TREATMENT...39

HOW DO I SURVIVE? 41
Basic Guidelines to Help..41
Keeping A Positive Attitude 41
Learn About Your Chosen Path 41
Build Support From Friends and Family 42
Be Responsible For Your Health Care 42
Follow Your Plans And Keep On Track 43
Give Back To Others 43

YOU HAVE RIGHTS AND RESPONSIBILITIES 45
Your Job is To Be An Educated Patient 45
Ask For Your Best Care 46
Be Treated With Respect 46
Make Informed and Educated Decisions........................47
Follow Your Agreed Treatment Plan...............................47

NEXT STEPS 49

Treatment Options For Kidney Disease and Failure

You have quite a few options with kidney failure. I know it might not feel like that right now. But when you reach a point of being in stage 5 kidney disease and you are severely affected by the side effects and symptoms of all the complications at that stage – next steps are something you should consider. By knowing what the options are before that time comes will create a sense of control in your life. You have control because you know what you have to choose from and what to decide on, and you can discuss it with your family or significant others.

Start With What You Can Do Now (You Are In Control)

Did I mention that you are in control? You might not feel like it, but you have the ability to choose your outcome. Mentally, you can decide what will happen. Physically, you will know what can happen. It might even change your commitment to your current diet and how you eat.

You ARE in control. You have choices. That is part of this book, to let you know what your choices are, but also to let you know there is still time. Even when you are looking dialysis square in the eyes, you can control your diet and slow the progression of kidney failure. Right now, you can learn more about your labs and diets (previous books) and make the changes you need to make to slow down kidney damage. Or you can choose to do nothing, and when your kidneys fail, you will make another choice. Make no mistake – choosing to do nothing is also a choice. Even after you start dialysis, you have more choices. You can change the type of dialysis you are on or even get a transplant.

AWARENESS

You probably already know that kidney disease is almost at epidemic proportions in our world. Almost one in 10 people have some kidney damage. They may not know it. And you are aware that you have some stage of kidney failure, but when did you find out? At stage 1 or stage 3? Probably stage 3! Now you need to kick it into high gear and find out what you can change.

Your awareness (knowledge, consciousness) about what causes kidney failure is key to stopping the progression of your own disease process. Knowing what foods to stop eating and what to eat more of are critical. As well as medications that affect – good or bad – your kidneys.

KNOWN RISK FACTORS

Early detection can lead to the ability to prevent further damage. You may or may not be aware of how you developed kidney failure. Risk factors affect how likely you are to get damage and control some of your ability to slow the disease. You can modify some risk factors and some you cannot.

Risk factors that you cannot modify are things like your age, gender, race and genetic makeup. As you age, you have a decline in kidney function that happens naturally and may or may not lead to you needing intervention. It seems that more African American persons develop kidney failure, and it is not clear why – but that is another risk factor that is not something you can change.

Risk factors that you can change are modifiable. These things can be changed over time and with assistance – so you should change them. The risk factors I am speaking of are: blood pressure level, blood sugar control, blood cholesterol levels, smoking, alcohol consumption, dietary intake, medication misuse, and weight. With kidney failure, you are encouraged to change the things that you can – slowly but surely. Review your medications with your doctor in light of your diagnosis. Talk about ways to lose the extra weight, and see if it helps with blood sugar control and blood pressure levels. They are related. Learn what your lab values are and how you can change them.

CONTROLLING YOUR RELATED DISEASES
When we review the things that we can do – one of the biggest ones is to control the diseases that are related to your kidney function. Your related diseases are diabetes and heart disease and you want to slow down the damage they are causing to your kidneys.

Diabetes should be controlled well and you should keep your HgA1c below 7.5% to have the most positive impact. When your blood sugars are high all the time, your blood cells are damaged. The damage they endure affects your kidneys because they flow through very small blood capillaries inside the kidneys when your body is cleaning the blood. The blood cells become misshapen and damage your kidneys. Kidneys have millions of small filters, so it can take some time to create enough damage to show up in your lab work. Once you know it's a problem, you need to keep your diabetes under control and checking your diet and blood sugars is a key.

Keeping your blood pressure low and in control is the other key to slowing the progression of the disease. Very similar to what happens in the kidneys when you have diabetes, when your blood pressure is too high – it causes damage in the small blood vessels as well. This is one of the reasons why your physician will have you take blood pressure lowering medication even if you don't have "high" blood pressure – it seems to help slow the progression of the disease. If you have high blood pressure, you should aim to have it at a level of 130/90 mmHg if you have diabetes or heart disease, and 140/90 mmHg if you have no related problems. [if your doctor wants it at a different level, listen to them]

MEDICATIONS AFFECT YOUR KIDNEYS
You might have thought about the medications you take as only those prescribed to you through your doctor. That is not the case. I would argue that food is also medication, but even if you don't think of food as a medication – all your herbs, vitamins, over the counter medications, shots and prescription medications are potentially affecting your kidneys. When you take a medication, it is absorbed (eventually) into your blood stream so it can perform the intended purpose. But your body has a method to deal with medications which are considered foreign to your system. Many drugs are removed from your blood and body through the kidneys. So, your medications affect your kidneys because they may damage the small blood vessels in the filtration process.

You might need to have a dose adjusted or change a medication completely. Talk to your doctor about medications and remind them you have kidney failure. Some medication doses may need to be changed, some adjusted and some stay the same. Many people with kidney failure should stop using NSAID's (non-steroidal anti-inflammatory drugs) like ibuprofen because of the potential for damage to the kidneys. Herbal supplements are not regulated and I would caution you that taking any is a risk. You should ensure you let your doctor know all the medications you take.

That said, your doctor may add some medications to help slow and control your kidney failure. Many times they add the ACE or ARB inhibitors (heart/blood pressure medications) that will lower blood pressure. They may change some things around so that your medications are doing the most good.

CHANGES AND PREVENTION

Your current status as a kidney patient means that you might be looking at how long until you become a dialysis patient, or hoping that you can avoid it all together. You need to make some changes to your life to slow down the progression of your disease.

TALK TO YOUR DOCTOR ABOUT YOUR LABS

Labs are a very critical part of your care. You should have a copy of the latest lab results when you leave the doctor's office. And track them over time to see if they are getting better or getting worse. If they continue to decline, start asking more specific questions about what you need to change to make the labs get better. Maybe you need to dig a little deeper into your motivation to get where you need to go. Know what labs are and what they mean – because they tell you a lot about where your disease is going and how fast.

CHANGE MEDICATIONS IF NEEDED

Medications, as mentioned before, are something that can affect your kidneys either positively or negatively (or not at all). You want to change your medications or dosages as your kidney failure progresses to ensure you are not taking too much or hurting your kidneys more. And go over your medications at every doctor visit to ensure you have not changed something that they need to address. Did a certain medication make you feel different from normal – ask! People don't realize it but as your kidneys stop filtering your blood as well, more of some medications remain in your system longer so you might need a lower dose.

FOLLOW A HEALTHY LOW PROTEIN DIET AND MEAL PATTERN

Eating healthy is all about knowing what you need and how much you need. Making a meal plan is key to being successful with eating right and sticking to your necessary limitations. When you are eating healthy for a kidney diet – it might not be the same as you are used to for a normal diet.

Eating a lower protein diet before you are on dialysis keeps your kidneys healthy longer. The protein breaks down into waste products and your kidneys have to handle them. It's much easier to help your kidneys out before you have too many problems. Spread out your protein through the day. Formulate a plan and stick to it. It gets easier with time.

EXERCISE – HOW EVER MUCH YOU CAN
You may be thinking – I am tired! I can't exercise. You might be right. Ask your doctor. But if you can do a few things – like get a chair aerobics CD and just sit in your chair and do them. You will make progress and eventually add on time and add on changes – resistance or other activities – that help you to build even more strength.

Exercise is something that we feel better once we start doing it, and maybe don't even like it when we are doing it, but once it's over we are sure it was the right thing to do. I assure you – starting small is the key. Walk around the block tonight. Walk a little further tomorrow. It all builds. Find a way and a time that you will do it and that you will be consistent with.

TRACK YOUR PROGRESS
Knowing where you started and where you are is critical to understanding what difference the changes you have made are doing for your body. If you have been able to stabilize at stage 3 for the last year by following a healthy diet, it's

important to feel good about that and not be upset by a small setback.

Use the information in your labs and from your doctor to know where you are and how you can improve. Document when you change something – like medications, or diet, or exercise – so you can determine what the catalyst was for the adjustment in your results. You could stay at stage 3 kidney failure for years with healthy habits, but sometimes your body has other ideas.

Seek Out Information For Yourself

You are your own best advocate. And having the knowledge that you need to ask the right questions is key. Know what each provider can do for you and your kidney disease, then ask them for help when you need it. Understand your health care allowances and rules so you can ask for what you need when you need it.

Be Your Own Advocate

Ask for the labs that you need to understand your condition. If your doctor says you should be ok and just come back another time – ask more questions if you don't like the answer.

Doctors sometimes are in a hurry. That does not make it ok for them to not tell you something, but you have to know what you need and what you are entitled to. They are human and you have your own best interests at heart. They may have been taught that you just wait out kidney failure until it gets to dialysis – don't stand for that.

See the Right Doctor And Ask For Referrals If Necessary

What is the right doctor? You usually have a "regular" doctor whom you work with on an ongoing basis. He or she might be a general practitioner or an internal medicine doctor. Either way, they are probably the one who diagnosed you (or ordered the labs) with kidney failure. Once you get diagnosed, you will go through treatment with them. But once you get to stage 3, you need to see a nephrologist. (kidney specific doctor). Learn more about what medications you are taking and have a longer talk with your general doctor – call and ask for a longer appointment so you can be comfortable asking questions.

What Can A Registered Dietitian Do?

Registered dietitians are the nutrition experts. They train in college and through internships to understand how food interacts with your disease state and make sure you are aware of the affects of foods. They can tell you foods to eat and not eat. And they can help you with a meal plan. They are good at analyzing your meals and helping you understand what part of your meals may be affecting your labs.

Nurses Know A Lot – Just Ask!

Think about it, the nephrologist's nurse sees patients just like you all day long. They take their vitals; ask them how they are doing. They hear about the struggles and successes that people have. They know what people do to fix their own problems. You should just ask them – "what do you think I should do?" Or "how do other patients handle this?" They can give you a few words of advice about how it usually works or tell your doctor to discuss it with you.

STAGES OF LOSS

Does it seem strange to talk about loss when you don't think you have lost anything? Well, this process is important to think through because you might not realize it now but you are on the verge of losing something very important – your kidney's function. Maybe you are in stage 3 and you don't think you will progress past that – great! But for many people, they do progress toward kidney failure – and knowing what to expect is helpful because the emotions can be overwhelming.

While these are the stage of grief or loss, you don't necessarily go through them at an even rate or even in the same order. But understanding and identifying them helps you deal with them better. They are not meant to be things to "get over" – these are feelings that are valid to experience.

DENIAL

Denial is the process of letting in only as much as we can handle. Maybe once your doctor says it's time for you to prepare for dialysis, you say to yourself – he's jumping the gun, I feel just fine. Or you try to figure out if you need another doctor to look at your labs and tell you it's ok.

This is your brain's way of processing the changes. You know what it means to start dialysis – time at the clinic 3 days a week or exchanges in peritoneal dialysis. But you think to yourself that it makes no sense. You are numb and probably don't want to talk about it. Think back to when you first learned that you had kidney failure – you didn't believe it! Not me!

ANGER

It goes from "not me!" to being angry that your doctor didn't tell you sooner. Lots of people write to me and say, "why didn't they tell me months ago?" You are so mad! And you have every right to be mad – feel your anger and let it be part of your healing. Sometimes the more angry you are the more motivated you are to make it right. But your anger helps you – it gives you direction to work on fixing something.

Along with the anger comes embarrassment. You are embarrassed that you have this health problem, and it's affecting your life. Now you have to get help, or have more doctor's appointments, or something else. Your personal shame is difficult to handle and may show up as anger.

BARGAINING

Now you begin to bargain. You may go through the "what if's" as well – what if you had found out sooner about the kidney problems, what if you had changed your diet, and what if you hadn't eaten so many oranges. If only you had done this or that. Maybe you bargain to devote your life to service and that will make this better.

You also feel like you can bargain with the pain. If you just tough it out, you will be ok. You might remain in this stage, trying to negotiate with a higher power or even yourself to make the problem go away.

DEPRESSION

You start to feel empty and hopelessness sets in. You are despondent, and not sure if you need to continue with this. You have tried to make changes and your body is fighting it, so why continue?

You might withdraw from friends and family a little, needing to try to understand what the next steps are – but probably not feeling like taking any of the next steps. It's normal to be depressed, and it's not a medical condition unless it continues for a long time or develops into harmful thoughts. You are losing something – time, energy, effort, to just begin with. It's a step to healing and understanding that you do have a purpose in life and you can make it through. As a matter of fact, by the time you start dialysis, you may very well be so lethargic that it will make you feel better and more active.

ACCEPTANCE

Acceptance does not mean that you are ok with the thought of dialysis, or you consider it your only option. At this point, you realize it's the best choice you have and you need to live with it for now. You might be on the transplant list, and hope to get a new kidney and this is temporary. Or you might know that you are starting with hemodialysis in a center but you plan to move to home hemodialysis as soon as you can. But this medical diagnosis is your new normal. And you can continue to fight it or you can work with it and make it your way.

So I encourage you to make it your way, to accept that it is going on and that you have to change. This doesn't mean that you won't ever be depressed about it again, because people move amongst the stages all the time. You are unique, and no one expects your path to be exactly like another person. But you need to know where you are headed, so we are going to talk about your options.

You are doing the right thing by searching out information prior to being placed on dialysis. Research shows that people lived longer (average of about 8 months) when they were educated prior to starting on dialysis about the things they need to do to have a healthier body once they started dialysis. If you plan your can have a better outcome.

WHAT OPTIONS DO I HAVE?

You might feel like your kidneys have the upper hand. I know you think you don't want to be on dialysis, and maybe you won't be. But studies show that knowing your options is one of the best ways you can regain control. You will understand what you need to do and what might happen.

Not all doctors agree on when you should start dialysis (at what point, or lab values) but know that as your kidney failure gets worse, you will feel worse. Many people dread the treatment, but find that once they have started on dialysis it was the best decision because they feel so much better. I encourage you to start talking about it early and understand what you can do. Know your options.

STAGE 5 ESRD

Stage 5 ESRD, or End Stage Renal Disease, is the condition in which your kidneys are no longer working (less than 10% function). At this point, you need to have artificial means to sustain your life, as your body is no longer able to filter your blood and keep you healthy. Your kidneys are probably not producing urine any longer. Your nephrologist and nurses should have prepared you for this.

WHAT DOES DIALYSIS DO?
Simply put, dialysis works as an artificial kidney to clean your blood. There are many types of dialysis, but they all try to do the same thing. They remove waste and excess water from your blood either through a machine or using your own body. The process involves something called dialysate which is a liquid that is used in dialysis. During dialysis, your blood passes through an area (either in your body or in a machine), and the dialysate is on the other side

of a barrier. The dialysate pulls the waste products out of your blood and into the solution, which is then discarded.

What happens is – your blood is on one side of a permeable membrane, and the "dialysate" is on the other side. As your blood passes by, the excess water and waste products are drawn into the dialysate. This is an imperfect process, and that is why when you are on dialysis you are able to eat a few more items and more protein – your body loses extra protein and minerals during dialysis. In addition, your artificial kidney is working more efficiently than your kidneys have been for a while.

PERITONEAL DIALYSIS

WHAT IS IT?

What is peritoneal dialysis (PD)? It is a process by which you place the dialysate in your abdominal cavity and it pulls the wastes from your blood. Once you have had the dialysate in your abdomen for a period of time, you drain the "used" solution and put in new solution. Research has shown that PD can keep your remaining kidney function longer. It is also gentler on the heart for people with heart problems.

It is a type of dialysis that can be done at home, and done continuously without using a machine. Let's start with talking about the name – peritoneal. Your peritoneum is a cavity that lines your abdomen and usually only contains a small amount of fluid. Dialysis solution (dialysate) can be placed into this cavity through a catheter and stays in the cavity in the abdomen. Your blood vessels pass near this cavity and allow the waste products in your blood to be removed. When you drain the "used" or waste fluid, these wastes are removed from your body. (I know it sounds complicated, but it's not.)

How Does It Work?

You might be wondering how the dialysate gets into the peritoneal cavity. Your doctor makes a small incision in your belly and inserts the catheter. Most of the tubes are placed near the belly button, but you should talk it through with your doctor. Once the tube is placed, it can take a few weeks to heal, but then it is ready. You will then do your exchanges – which is the process of removing the used fluid and putting in clean fluid so that your dialysis is done over the day or night.

There are several types of peritoneal dialysis that are options.

CAPD

CAPD stands for continuous ambulatory peritoneal dialysis. This means that it is done "all the time". After about 4 hours, the fluid has done what it can and should be exchanged. You may do 3-5 exchanges during the day and that can take about 30 minutes. You must be careful when doing exchanges to avoid getting an infection. Because you have dialysis going on all the time, you have very few fluid and food restrictions.

CCPD

You might not be able to do exchanges at work or need more blood cleaning than CAPD can provide. CCPD stands for continuous cycling peritoneal dialysis. This process uses a machine to do a lot of exchanges at night while you are sleeping, and may eliminate or cut down on the amount of exchanges required during the day.

WHAT DOES IT REQUIRE?

This system requires you to do a lot of the work of your own care. It is your responsibility to do the exchanges and hook up the machine. You can do it while traveling but it does require equipment in your home. You also may have large amounts of dialysate in your house so you can do the exchanges which might affect you and the amount of storage you have.

It can be best for people who are able to do the exchanges independently. If you want to maintain some variety and flexibility PD can help you do that. You will still be able to travel and use PD, plus it requires less time at the clinic or doctor's office. You have to do a very clean exchange and ensure you are using the proper procedure.

If you feel a little queasy about doing exchanges just reading this, you might not be the best candidate. There are no needles in this process.

GOOD THINGS ABOUT PD

- You have fewer diet restrictions since it is done all the time
- You usually feel the same all the time, not ups and downs
- You are in control and manage the exchanges yourself
- You have flexibility to work the exchanges around your work day
- No needles are used in the process
- No blood is usually seen, and it's generally painless
- You can travel or do PD at a variety of locations
- You can take part in your normal activities including work

- It's gentle on your heart

BAD THINGS ABOUT PD
- You might feel bloated all the time with the fluid in your abdomen
- You may need extra protein in your diet
- Dialysate has sugar in it and can affect diabetes patients
- You have to use specific procedures to reduce the chance of infections
- You feel like you are doing dialysis all the time, even on vacation
- You might not like having a catheter in your abdomen
- You might have some pain while the catheter incision is healing
- PD supplies take up a lot of storage space and the boxes are heavy
- PD works best for smaller people, and may be best if you have some kidney function left
- You may be restricted in some activities to reduce the chance of infection
- You might gain weight from the fluid and sugar in the dialysate adding calories to your body

HEMODIALYSIS

The most common treatment used to treat advanced and permanent kidney disease is hemodialysis (HD). Hemo – meaning blood, and dialysis – cleaning. So you are allowing a small part of your blood to be outside of your body during treatment to be cleaned.

WHAT IS IT?
Hemodialysis is a process through which a machine takes blood from your body and sends it through a dialyzer (a special type of filter). Either you go to a center or you can do it at home. It does require you to spend some "quiet" time not being too active and sitting in a chair. It usually is done 3 days a week, although with home HD you can do it more often. Research has shown that more often is probably better (since your kidneys worked 24/7 – best to mimic their process). Many people find that they are tired or worn out by the process, more so with in-center dialysis.

Much of the time patients may feel that dialysis will limit them, but they find that the process makes them feel much better and they have a better quality of life than they have had for a long time due to the ill effects of poorly functioning kidneys.

HOW DOES IT WORK?
HD works by taking about 1 cup of blood at a time (you have about 10 in your blood) and sending it through the machine. The dialyzer is a large filter. The inside contains thousands of fibers through which your blood flows. The dialysate flows around the fibers and brings the wastes out of the blood. The machines are about the size of a large TV and reside on a stand. Removing the excess water and waste materials from your blood serves to control your

blood pressure and keep the proper balance of potassium and sodium in your body.

HD can take about 3-5 hours to clean your blood. You will likely have a restricted diet – mainly fluids but also some potassium. Between dialysis days you have to stick very closely to the diet so you don't feel poorly.

People often worry about the needles used, and the process does involve needles. You may learn to insert them yourself, and that may make it hurt less. You can also use numbing cream to keep the pain down. Your doctors often need to create an access line, called a fistula, which has to heal prior to use. A fistula is a connection between an artery and a vein, and is usually started prior to dialysis treatment beginning so you have the best type of access.

IN CENTER HD
In center HD is the most common type of dialysis, and many people think it's the only type of dialysis. Most people start at a center, and you may determine that is the best type of treatment for you. Once you have the "hang" of it, you can do much of the process yourself even in a center.

What this involves is going to a dialysis center 3 days per week. Usually Monday, Wednesday and Friday or Tuesday, Thursday and Saturday. You might come for a morning, afternoon or evening shift. You are usually there 3-5 hours – including time waiting for a machine, getting hooked up and letting the dialysis machine do it's work.

You can learn to insert your own needles, take your blood pressure, set up the machine and get it started. You will have the staff there if you have a problem, but you can be self sufficient and yet still be in a controlled environment that will keep you feeling "safe".

HOME HD

If you can operate a car, you can perform your own dialysis at home. You will need training that lasts several weeks, but you can have a great deal of independence once you have mastered the process.

You have the machine at home, and most of the time you have to have a "helper" person (Family or home health worker) who assists you. But the process of having it at home allows you to use the machine for longer, which makes for better dialysis (remember your kidneys work 24/7). Some of the machines are portable, and can be taken on a car ride or on a plane, allowing you to travel. You don't have to purchase the machine: it is provided as part of your care.

The main differences are that you have a person standing by via phone and you do a lot of the work yourself. But many people like it because they can live a little further away from a dialysis center. You do have to store the equipment and solutions in your home, taking up storage space.

WHAT DOES IT REQUIRE?

Either way, hemodialysis requires you to spend 3-6 hours sitting or lying down and being "tied" to a machine. It may require more time. You will need transportation to the center, or be able to hook up the machine on your own.

You will also require a surgery to get a fistula put in, so planning ahead is important once you know that you will need dialysis. Most people feel much better once starting

HD and even though it's inconvenient for them to have to go to a center – the reward of feeling much better is worth it.

If you are able to do some self care, the staff will often let you do as much as you are able, giving you a level of freedom. People often report that the needle sticks don't hurt quite as much when you do them yourself.

GOOD THINGS ABOUT HD
- You don't have to think about dialysis all the time – it's a structured time
- You can have nurses do most of the care for you, or you can learn to do it yourself
- You have set aside free time to work on quiet activities, read, write or study
- It can be a social experience to go to a center and meet the other patients and staff
- You can learn to monitor the machine yourself and take care of your own dialysis at home if you want to
- You can plan ahead and take trips with either type of dialysis
- You can do most of your usual activities
- You don't have a stomach full of fluid all the time
- You feel good once the treatment is done
- You can be in your own home if you choose and have family around you
- You don't have to drive to a center for Home HD
- With Home HD your diet can be more normal if you are able to do treatments more often than 3 times per week.

BAD THINGS ABOUT HD

- Your meal plan is much more rigid on in center HD because you have limited time on the dialysis machine
- Nurses are taking care of many people at one time during the in center HD so you might not get someone to come over right away if it's not an emergency
- The treatment schedule might not fit your life, and you might have to drive a way to get to a center.
- Two needle sticks with large needles are used during treatments
- You might feel "washed out" right after dialysis
- Between treatments you might not feel very good because of the lack of filtration of your blood allows waste products to build up
- You have to go to the treatments or do them at home.
- You might spend a lot of time setting up the machine, getting it ready and using it with home HD.
- You may have to store large amounts of equipment with home HD
- You will need to get training with home HD so you can perform the steps yourself and have a partner assist you

TRANSPLANT

Some people with kidney disease look at transplant as a cure. But it really is just another treatment. It may be a fairly good treatment, but it still requires work and some major life changes as well.

WHAT IS IT?
Transplant is when you receive a new kidney and doctors place it into your body, and connect the blood and ureter to your body. The new kidney functions in the same way as your other kidneys did when they were healthy.

You might receive a kidney from a family member or non-family member willing to donate. This is called a living donation. People can live with one kidney, and in fact, your kidney can enlarge and take over much of the needed function. So it's possible to have a kidney transplanted from a living donor who is willing to go through the donation process.

You also could receive a kidney from a person who is deceased and matches your blood type. In this case, you will be on a list and be waiting from weeks to years for a matching kidney. During that time, you might be on dialysis while you wait.

HOW DOES IT WORK?
Transplantation requires surgery to remove the kidney from a living donor, and surgery to place the kidney in the recipient. The surgery is 3-4 hours and you must be ready to go on a moment's notice when you get the call about being a match for a deceased donor's kidney.

Unfortunately, there are not enough donors for all of those people waiting for kidneys. You are encouraged to ask family to see if they are a match. You will be on dialysis while you wait, and the new kidney requires some special treatment.

A new kidney could be rejected by your body. You will need to take medications to prevent it from being rejected that may subject you to other illnesses. Most of the time, you will need to follow some limitations in your diet (mainly a low sodium diet), and take your medications daily. Kidneys can last for a long time once transplanted, or they can be rejected after many years. For the most part, about 80% of people do pretty well once they have a transplant.

WHAT DOES IT REQUIRE?
Getting a new kidney requires a few things. You might have a living family member who is willing to donate their kidney. The living donor's cost will be covered by Medicare, so they will not have to pay for the surgery. You will get surgery at the same time, and you can spend 2-3 weeks recovering from the surgery. It is an abdominal surgery, and will need some time to heal.

If you have to wait for a donor kidney on the donation list, the time could be from a few months to a few years. You might have to travel to get the kidney last minute, but you will be able to benefit from the kidney working inside you and no longer having to do dialysis for as long as the kidney works.

GOOD THINGS ABOUT TRANSPLANT
- Once the kidney starts working, you will not have to do dialysis
- After you heal from the surgery, you won't have to spend 12-15 hours doing dialysis

- Your fluid limitations will be removed since you have a working kidney
- You may be able to work full time and stay more active
- You may be able to take part in your usual activities
- You can develop a strong bond with a family or friend who donated a kidney
- You should feel much better once the kidney starts working

BAD THINGS ABOUT TRANSPLANT
- Your body might reject the kidney and you will have to go back on dialysis (or never stop)
- You have to take the drugs to keep your body from rejecting the kidney daily, and they can be costly and cause other problems
- You will need to drink plenty of water to keep hydrated and eat a low salt diet
- It is major surgery to get your transplant and will require recovery time
- You will be limited from playing contact sports where your kidney could be damaged
- You will not know how long you will have to wait for a deceased donor kidney

No Treatment

For a group of people who may be seriously ill, and dialysis would not add to the quality of life, the option to not pursue treatment is available. While it is not for everyone, it's important to realize it is a choice. You should know that it exists.

You may be at the end of life, or with someone who is at the end of life, and feels that they would prefer to not do treatment.

Realize, this choice means that you will be preparing for "palliative care" which is the term used for keeping someone comfortable and free of pain as they prepare of a peaceful and meaningful passing. This choice should not be made lightly, and should be the product of discussion with professionals about the options and potential outcomes.

This option is really only for those who will likely not gain improvement in quality of life by participating in dialysis. While people may sometimes feel hopeless or depressed, that is not the same as nearing end of life.

How Do I Survive?

This is a big life change you will be going through, whether you choose PD or HD and eventually get a transplant. It is not the end of the world, it's a new chapter!

Basic Guidelines to Help

We spoke at the beginning of this book about the stages of loss or grief. Understanding that you will go through several stages and knowing what might happen can be a good way to deal with it. But sometimes you are in the midst of anger and you don't know how to handle it – you are just angry and you want to be angry!

Here are a few suggestions about how some simple changes in the way you approach life could help you with dealing with this huge life change. You will have challenges, both with kidney disease, and in other parts of your life. You can get through them with a little help.

Keeping A Positive Attitude

"Whether you think you can or you think you can't, you're right" Henry Ford

That statement may or may not be profound to you, but it makes a great point about how attitude changes the way we approach things and ultimately the outcomes we receive from the things we do. Staying positive will help you overcome when things do seem too difficult. You will see the hope instead of the darkness.

Learn About Your Chosen Path

What you have done by going through this book is important. Now that you know what your choices are, you will increase your patience and calm your fears. Knowing what is to come, and what you can do to avoid it, are invaluable. It makes you less afraid of what is to come, and helps your doctors because you are being proactive about your care.

BUILD SUPPORT FROM FRIENDS AND FAMILY
Your friends and family may not understand what you are going through. Or they may say they understand but it's a hard road and they can't know unless you tell them. Your health care providers will be there to explain some things about your care. But others can be there emotionally and with other types of support – driving you to appointments or bringing you a meal when you are sick.

Talking about what you are going through can be helpful. You might be having an angry spell, and it's hard to like someone when they are negative and fatalistic. Take a moment to talk to someone who will listen. And avoid those who are negative or bring you down. If they are constantly complaining or making you feel bad about what you are doing, you have a need to avoid that toxicity because it will bring you down as well.

BE RESPONSIBLE FOR YOUR HEALTH CARE
In this book, we talked a little about how you can do a lot of your care on your own. It is important to realize that you are in charge and you are responsible for your own care. Being a victim will get you nothing – feeling like you are being punished or can't control your life won't help. You have to follow through, no one can do it for you.

Take an active role. Learn about what you can do to stop kidney failure from progressing. Ask appropriate questions of your doctors. Know your labs. Eat a healthy diet.

Follow Your Plans And Keep On Track

Work with your doctor to determine which plan is the best for you to follow. You shouldn't be passive about it, learn what you need to learn. Start the process to get your fistula when it's time.

The more consistent you are in your treatment, the better your outcomes. You will get the best treatment when you know what you need. You will be more hopeful about the future when you are doing the things that you have decided to pursue with passion.

Give Back To Others

While it may seem strange, often we get lost in our own worlds of hurt and don't see that others are hurting as well. Volunteering or helping out others in your same situation can be a good way to understand how you are doing and helping others always makes you feel better.

Sometimes you might be able to help someone decide on the right treatment for them. Sometimes you could just be a good listener to the person and know where they are coming from. Either way, keep from getting lost in your own sorrows by helping others.

You Have Rights and Responsibilities

You may have many rights as a patient. Part of having rights is also having responsibilities. It's how you use your rights and take care of your responsibilities that makes the difference. It's like a job that you have to advocate for yourself. But when you advocate for yourself, you have much better outcomes and less stress since you know that you made an informed decision about it.

Your Job is To Be An Educated Patient

Yes, I said job. You have to know your rights to parts of your medical records and how decisions are made. And to participate in that decision making process for your health. You should know what the best sources for you are related to your care and what is to come and how you can manage it. Don't feel like you do not have choices – ask them what they are.

Specifically, you have a right to know what is wrong with you and what your options are. If you have stage 5 kidney failure, and your options are similar to what we discussed in this book, you know where to start choosing. You need to know what services your clinic offers and what you are eligible for – and if you can do any of the additional things by yourself.

You also have a right to know how much care will cost and how you can pay for it. Your clinic might have rules about how you can pay, but you can sometimes talk to the manager and work out a deal if you need it. You should also be informed of the way to file a complaint, and how to get a copy of an Advanced Medical Directive. Finally, you should also know that you can get a copy of the chart they record your information on and how they write the notes.

You should advocate for yourself and make sure you have a plan for care. Whether it's before you start on dialysis or now that you have been on dialysis – know what the goals of treatment are. Know what your doctor thinks they should do to make you better, and how much "better" you might get.

Ask For Your Best Care

Once you know what care you can receive – whether it be hemodialysis, peritoneal dialysis or other options, you should make sure your doctor manages that. If they do not, consider going to another provider. Your doctor is required to tell you about treatment options even if they don't provide it at that clinic, so ask questions.

You should go to the library to learn more when you need to know certain things. It's your life and you have a right to the treatment you want. You should know your insurance and be able to understand what part of the care you will be responsible to pay for. You can possibly get some help with bills, but the first step is knowing what they are so you can make any changes that you can as an option.

Be Treated With Respect

You should be treated with respect. Many times we feel disrespected in some way – whether it is by a nurse, or another provider. Standing up for yourself is fine, just don't attack other people. One of the things that people often don't think about related to respect is that your caregivers wash their hands before they start treatment with you. That is tantamount – and you should ask if you don't see them doing it.

You can go a long way with respect by saying please and thank you. It might seem odd, but the little things matter.

Yelling, making threats and being violent toward staff is a good way to get removed from a clinic, not the way to get your best care.

MAKE INFORMED AND EDUCATED DECISIONS

You have a right to make a decision that is in your best interest. not your doctor's, or your clinic's or anyone else's. Yours and your family. If it's best for you to do PD because you want to continue to work – if you are capable of meeting the requirements to do that treatment – then you should do it.

You also have a right to know what is in your medical chart. You can request copies (there may be a procedure or forms) and ask your doctor's about things in your chart that they may have documented – like your treatment options, how sick you are, how likely you are to get better, and your lab tests. It's your medical information – if you want to know you can ask. You have a responsibility to be truthful about your condition and answer all questions to the best of your ability to allow yourself to get the best care possible. Remind your doctor that you have diabetes, for example, when they are prescribing medications.

You can change doctors or ask for second opinions if you don't agree with the plan your doctor has for you. It's important that you are on the same page. You might transfer to another clinic if you feel they are not giving you the best care. But give them a chance to understand your concerns before you get too upset and they will likely fix the problems.

FOLLOW YOUR AGREED TREATMENT PLAN

Once you agree to a treatment plan with your doctor, you have an obligation to follow it to the best of your ability.

You should come to your appointments on time, with your information about changes and any side effects you have noticed. You should be ready to ask questions about changes and things that you need to know about. You need to be doing the treatments your doctor prescribes – medications, dialysis, and nutrition.

You also need to stay active – as much as you can. You may have heart or diabetes problems, and you need to stay as healthy as you can. Show your doctors and nurses that you are genuinely interested in your care, and they will work with you to make the struggle less stressful.

NEXT STEPS

1. After you have read through this book, ask yourself which program seems to be the best one for you. Think through the good and bad things and how important they are for you.
2. Once you reach the stage of kidney failure that requires you to start on dialysis, you now understand that you have choices. And no matter where you are now, you can change.
3. If you are on dialysis, know that if something is not working well for you, it's time to have a discussion with your doctor about changes.
4. Consider if you are doing what you can to advocate for your own care and do as much as you can to help yourself. See what else you can do by speaking with a nurse in your clinic about what is available.